Foods 33+   Mayes

THE BIBLE CURE® FOR

MENOPAUSE

D0972543

DON COLBERT, M.D.

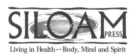

Living in Health—Body, Mind and Spirit

THE BIBLE CURE FOR MENOPAUSE
by Don Colbert, M.D.
Published by Siloam Press
A part of Strang Communications Company
600 Rinehart Road
Lake Mary, Florida 32746
www.creationhouse.com

This book or parts thereof may not be reproduced
in any form, stored in a retrieval system or transmit-
ted in any form by any means—electronic, mechani-
cal, photocopy, recording or otherwise—without
prior written permission of the publisher, except as
provided by United States of America copyright law.

Unless otherwise noted, all Scripture quotations are
from the Holy Bible, New Living Translation, copyright © 1996, Tyndale House Publishers, Inc.,
Wheaton, Illinois 60189.

Scripture quotations marked NKJV are from the New
King James Version of the Bible. Copyright © 1979,
1980, 1982 by Thomas Nelson, Inc., publishers.
Used by permission.

Copyright © 2000 by Don Colbert, M.D.
All rights reserved

Library of Congress Catalog Card Number: 99-85845
International Standard Book Number: 0-88419-683-6

This book is not intended to provide medical advice or to take the place of medical advice and treatment from your personal physician. Readers are advised to consult their own doctors or other qualified health professionals regarding the treatment of their medical problems. Neither the publisher nor the author takes any responsibility for any possible consequences from any treatment, action or application of medicine, supplement, herb or preparation to any person reading or following the information in this book. If readers are taking prescription medications, they should consult with their physicians and not take themselves off of medicines to start supplementation without the proper supervision of a physician.

02 03 04 05   10 9 8 7 6
Printed in the United States of America

A Brand-New
Season of Your Life

A woman's life is filled with the joy of many wonderful seasons, according to a wise Creator's design. The Word of God says, "To everything there is a season, a time for every purpose under heaven" (Eccles. 3:1, NKJV).

In the springtime, a woman's femininity awakens in the tender bloom of her youth. In the summer, her fruitful body fills her life with the busy joy of babies and children. But the autumn of a woman's life can be the most wonderful season of all. During the years of menopause, a harvest of all the good things a woman has planted into those around her comes back to her. In addition, the joy of grownup children, grandchildren and the freedom of new pursuits can paint her life with a burst of change as beautiful and as varied as a dazzling display of autumn color.

If you have entered into the autumn season of menopause, you are probably sensing that you are embarking upon a special season of great change. And since new challenges always accompany change, you may be filled with questions. Don't be alarmed; it is all according to God's wonderful plan for your life. Look at this powerful promise in Scripture:

> "For I know the plans I have for you," says the LORD. "They are plans for good and not for disaster, to give you a future and a hope."
>
> —JEREMIAH 29:11

God created your body to go through your life changes in a natural, healthy and positive way. My prayer for you as a result of reading and putting into practice what you need from this book is "that all is well with you and that your body is as healthy as I know your soul is" (3 John 2).

God's desire for you as you pass through the natural life transition of premenopause, menopause and postmenopause is to be healthy and renewed, as the psalmist declares, "He fills my life with good things. My youth is renewed like the eagle's!" (Ps. 103:5). You may feel that menopause signals an aging and deterioration of life. God's plan contradicts that! As you mature physically, God desires to renew your strength and vitality so that you feel young, strong and able to serve Him in all things.

What is menopause? It's neither a disease nor abnormality! It's simply the stopping or cessation of the monthly female menstrual cycle. Women who have not had a menstrual cycle for a year are considered postmenopausal.

In the United States, many women face menopause with fear and trepidation. About 50 percent of women in the United States experience some degree of significant symptoms during menopause.

So, as you read this book, get ready to feel better physically, emotionally and spiritually. This Bible Cure booklet is filled with practical steps, hope, encouragement and understanding on how to stay fit and healthy. In this book, you will

uncover God's divine plan of health
for body, soul and spirit
through modern medicine, good nutrition
and the medicinal power
of Scripture and prayer.

You will discover life-changing, healing scriptures throughout this booklet to help you focus on rising above menopause with God's help. As you read, apply and trust God's promises.

You will also uncover powerful Bible Cure prayers to help you line up your thoughts and feelings with God's plan of divine health for you—a plan that includes living victoriously instead of painfully. In this Bible Cure booklet, you will learn how to rise above menopause as you read the following chapters:

There is much you can do to prevent or overcome the symptoms of menopause. Now is the time to begin with a God-given plan that will give you the confidence, determination and knowledge to embrace the challenge of change with tranquility and calm. God's peace is greater than anything you now face. You can feel better physically, which will also positively impact all your relationships!

I pray that these practical suggestions for health, nutrition and fitness will bring wholeness and health to your life and relationships. May they deepen your relationship with God and further empower you to serve and worship Him.

—DON COLBERT, M.D.

A BIBLE CURE PRAYER
FOR YOU

*Heavenly Father, You have declared in
Your Word that You desire my strength to
be renewed as the eagle's. I claim Your
desire for me to prosper and be in good
health, both in body and soul. I need Your
strength to develop a positive attitude for
rising above menopause and its symptoms. By Your stripes I have been healed,
so I receive Your healing for any pain and
discomfort in my body during this transition time in my physical life process.
Thank You for caring for me and all my
feelings and emotions. Empower me to
make wise choices and follow the guide-
lines in Your Word concerning healthy
nutritional and lifestyle choices. By Your
Spirit, help me to pray in Your will that I
might know Your abundant life for myself
and in my relationships. Heal any hurt I
may have caused others when I have not
felt well. Thank You, Lord, for hearing and
answering my prayers so that I might fully
serve You—body, soul and spirit. Amen.*

Chapter 1

Understanding Your
Season of Change

G od intends for you to embrace your season of
change as a beautiful time in your life. For the
Bible says, "He has made everything beautiful in
its time [season]" (Eccles. 3:11, NKJV).

The good news about menopause is that it's the
natural, God-created pathway for you to mature
physically in your life. You are not sick, and your
symptoms can be controlled so that you can completely enjoy this time of your life. God has provided natural steps you can take through
nutrition, fitness and faith to pass through your
season of menopause with joy, peace, grace and
victory.

You are destined to have the upper hand over
any symptoms, discomfort or pain. God has

promised, "If you listen to these commands of the LORD your God and carefully obey them, the LORD will make you the head and not the tail, and you will always have the upper hand" (Deut. 28:13).

Getting the upper hand will take a little understanding about this special time of life.

Understanding Menopause

At birth there are about one million eggs in a woman's ovaries. That number drops to about three to four hundred thousand at puberty, but only about four hundred of these eggs will actually mature during her reproductive years. With each menstrual cycle, hundreds of eggs will be lost. When a woman no longer has any eggs left in her ovaries, she then stops menstruating and goes into menopause.

If you are going through menopause, you may be experiencing some of the following symptoms:

- Hot flashes
- Mood swings
- Frequent vaginal infections
- Cold hands and feet
- Night sweats
- Fatigue
- Headaches

- Decreased sex drive
- Breast tenderness
- Palpitations of the heart
- Insomnia
- Drying of the skin
- Vaginal itching
- Bladder infections
- Vaginal dryness
- Dizziness
- Inability to concentrate

The symptoms of menopause most frequently experienced include hot flashes and dryness of the vaginal lining, otherwise known as "atrophic vaginitis." As many as 80 percent of menopausal women experience some hot flashes. The hot flashes usually are the first sign that menopause is close at hand. During a hot flash blood vessels dilate and skin temperature rises and flushes the skin. This usually occurs about the head and neck and only lasts a few seconds to a minute. These symptoms may be associated with headaches, dizziness, a rapid heartbeat and fatigue.

For the majority of women, menopause occurs at about fifty years of age. However, it can occur as early as thirty-five or forty, and may occur as late as fifty-five or sixty years of age. The period of time before menopause is known as the perimenopause period, and the period of time after menopause is known as the postmenopausal period.

Many women in their twenties and thirties have gone through a surgical menopause due to the removal of their ovaries. If you have had a hysterectomy and your ovaries removed, then you will also go into menopause, and the symptoms may be quite severe. But if you will take the physical and spiritual steps described in this book,

> So I tell you, don't worry about everyday life—whether you have enough food, drink, and clothes. Doesn't life consist of more than food and clothing? Look at the birds. They don't need to plant or harvest or put food in barns because your heavenly Father feeds them. And you are far more valuable to him than they are.
> —MATTHEW 6:25–26

you can rise above menopause to a strong, vital life without discomfort and pain.

Premenopause

Premenopause (also called perimenopause) often begins in a woman's midthirties. If a woman does not ovulate, then her body does not produce adequate amounts of progesterone. Thus she becomes deficient in this hormone, which leads to having a large amount of estrogen and a very small amount of progesterone, a condition otherwise known as "estrogen dominance."

A BIBLE CURE HEALTH TIP

Are You Experiencing These Symptoms of Premenopause?

- ❑ Fatigue
- ❑ Loss of sex drive
- ❑ Irritability
- ❑ Depression
- ❑ Cold hands and feet
- ❑ Night sweats
- ❑ Craving for carbohydrates and sweets
- ❑ Fatigue upon arising in the morning, leading to caffeine addiction

- ❑ Weight gain
- ❑ Mood swings
- ❑ Headaches
- ❑ Low metabolic rate
- ❑ Hot flashes

Women often arrive at a physician's office because of fatigue, mood swings, loss of sex drive and depression. Many doctors prescribe Prozac or another type of antidepressant for these women. But what their bodies really need is the hormone progesterone.

Ovulation is simply the release of a mature egg from the ovarian follicle. Menstrual cycles can continue for years without the woman ovulating, but she will not be producing adequate progesterone. She will, however, continue to produce sufficient amounts—sometimes too much—estrogen. As a result, many women begin to gain weight and develop water retention and bloating along with irritability and mood swings.

These symptoms are only the beginning of perimenopause. It is rather common during the perimenopausal period that estrogen levels will rise significantly, leading to quite heavy periods. This leads to breast tenderness, water retention, weight gain and extreme moodiness.

Your Changing Hormones

At menopause, the fall of the hormone progesterone is much greater than the fall of estrogen. The estrogen falls about 40 to 60 percent. However, the progesterone level decline is nearly twelve times greater. The pituitary gland responds to this drop in both estrogen and progesterone by increasing secretion of the hormones FSH and LH. These two hormones cause the ovaries and adrenal glands to secrete more male-type hormones called *androgens*, which can lead to growth of facial hair, obesity, thinning of the hair and other unpleasant side effects. These androgens are also converted to estrogens, which can lead to increased fat cells in the hips, thighs, abdomen and buttocks.

You may be experiencing some of these effects already. But take heart, God has created a number of natural and spiritual ways to combat these negative effects.

Your Monthly Cycles

In order to fully understand menopause, you need to understand the menstrual cycle. Menstruation is simply the monthly vaginal flow of blood. At the beginning of the menstrual cycle the uterus prepares a thickened lining in preparation for a pregnancy. If the egg is not fertilized, this lining will be shed, and a new lining will be prepared. This monthly occurrence is due mainly to the interaction of the hormones estrogen and progesterone.

In the first week after menstruation, estrogen is the dominant hormone, which causes a buildup of the lining of your uterus. Estrogen also stimulates the ovarian follicles to develop an egg in preparation for fertilization. Ovulation occurs when the ovarian follicle releases the mature egg. Once the egg is released, the follicle becomes a corpus luteum. The corpus luteum then begins to produce the other female hormone, progesterone, during the second half of the menstrual cycle. The progesterone causes the uterine lining to mature, getting the lining ready for a fertilized egg.

At the time of ovulation, when the progesterone rises there is also a rise in body temperature, usually one degree Fahrenheit. If fertilization of the egg does not occur, then the estrogen and progesterone levels will fall rapidly, thus causing shedding of the lining of the uterus, resulting in menstrual flow.

> *I know how to live on almost nothing or with everything. I have learned the secret of living in every situation, whether it is with a full stomach or empty, with plenty or little. For I can do everything with the help of Christ who gives me the strength I need.*
> —PHILIPPIANS 4:12–13

However, if pregnancy does occur, the progesterone level will increase, which will thus preserve the lining of the uterus for the developing embryo. Your menstrual cycle is dependent upon these two hormones—estrogen and progesterone.

However, two other hormones from the pituitary

gland also affect your menstrual cycle: FSH and LH. FSH is a follicle-stimulating hormone, triggering the ovary to produce estrogen. FSH also causes the ovarian follicle that houses the egg to mature.

LH is the other hormone in the pituitary. This hormone triggers ovulation by rising rapidly, usually a day prior to ovulation. LH then rapidly falls once progesterone is secreted by the follicle corpus luteum.

LH and FSH are under the control of a portion of the brain called the *hypothalamus*. The hypothalamus sends a hormone to the pituitary gland, called gonadotropin-releasing hormone. This hormone causes the release of FSH and LH, which are gonadotropins from the pituitary gland.

As you can see, the fairly complicated system of menopause depends on hormonal messengers from the hypothalamus, pituitary and ovaries. Now that I have described the basic menstrual cycle, I want to help you understand in more detail the two main hormones—estrogen and progesterone.

How Does Estrogen Affect My Body?

Progesterone and estrogen are two of the steroid hormones in the body. Most people think there is just one form of estrogen in the body. However, there are actually three forms of estrogen in the body. There are also different types of estrogen compounds outside of the body. These include plant estrogens and xenoestrogens.

The three estrogens in the body are estrone, estriol and estradiol. *Estrone* is produced in the ovaries and in the fatty tissues. *Estriol* is made by the placenta or by the adrenal glands and is usually made from the hormone DHEA. During pregnancy estriol is the main source of estrogen and is produced by the placenta. Estradiol and estrone are present only in very small amounts. *Estradiol,* which is made by the ovaries, is one thousand times more potent in its stimulating effect to the breast as compared to estriol. Estriol is not nearly as stimulating to the breast, but is very beneficial to the cervix, vagina and vulva by preventing vaginal dryness, itching and discomfort during intercourse.

During menopause, the body begins to produce less and less of the estrogens that you need. However, there are other estrogen-like compounds found in that environment. Some are phytoestrogens. These come from plants, and they have weak estrogen-like activity. However, they compete for the same estrogen receptors in the body.

Good News

In the next chapter we will discover the God-created natural estrogens that will help your body rise above the negative symptoms of menopause. The good news is that God has provided all that you need to go through the natural, physical transition of menopause with comfort, ease and much less irritability. Discover what works best for you as an individual through these Bible Cure steps of natural substances, good nutrition, vitamins and supplements.

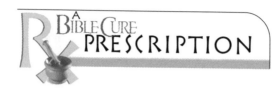

R A BIBLE CURE
PRESCRIPTION

Write out a prayer in your own words to ask God
for wisdom and direction to apply the wisdom
and knowledge you are receiving from this book:

_____

_____

_____

_____

_____

_____

_____

_____

_____

_____

_____

_____

Chapter 2

Embracing Change
With Natural Hormones

S cripture teaches us how God created plants for our benefit. Psalm 104:14 says:

> You cause grass to grow for the cattle.
> You cause plants to grow for people to
> use. You allow them to produce food
> from the earth.

God has created remarkable, natural substances to help your body overcome the uncomfortable symptoms of menopause. As you know already, the estrogen hormones in your body begin to decrease during menopause. God has made phytoestrogens available in plants to supplement your body's supply of needed estrogens.

The very plants that God created will help you

to rise above menopause so that you feel better and are able to serve God more fully.

The Promise of Phytoestrogens

Hollywood screenwriter Christine Conrad, age fifty-four and author of *Natural Women, Natural Menopause,* defines plant-derived hormones as "natural" and implies that Premarin, which comes from horses, is not.[1] Under the care of her naturopathic physician and coauthor, Marcus Laux, Conrad claims to have safely and comfortably navigated her own menopause, which followed a hysterectomy she underwent at age forty-six. "The natural hormones," she says, "don't have side effects". . . . To be sure, phytoestrogens look promising. Wake Forest University epidemiologist Dr. Gregory Burke has launched a clinical trial designed to measure the effects of soy phytoestrogens on 280 perimenopausal women. Already, he says, the results of a smaller, preliminary trial suggest that the estrogenic compounds soy contains—genistein and diadzein—relieve the severity of hot flashes and also lower cholesterol. But promising as it seems, cautions Burke, no

14

one yet knows whether soy can provide what women want—all the benefits of Premarin without its negative effects.[2]

The Problem
With Standard Treatments

Too often, doctors treat menopause as a disease instead of a natural, God-created life transition. They prescribe medications to treat the symptoms instead of helping your body overcome those symptoms naturally. The usual drugs prescribed are Premarin and Provera.

✓ A Bible Cure HealthFact

Premarin—Menopause as a natural, physical life transition has symptoms of hot flashes that occur in up to 80 percent of women. However, physicians treat menopause as a disease, and synthetic hormones are used as hormonal replacement therapy. Premarin is the most common estrogen hormone prescription written in America. Premarin actually contains estrogens that are derived from the urine of pregnant mares.

Provera—The other hormone commonly

prescribed with Premarin is Provera. Provera is a synthetic form of progesterone and is commonly taken in conjunction with Premarin in order to prevent cancer of the uterus. Unfortunately, these synthetic hormones cause water retention and excessive accumulation of fat, especially in the abdomen, hips, thighs and breasts. Even though Premarin and Provera help to prevent uterine cancer, they do not prevent breast or ovarian cancer. In fact, estrogen actually fuels these cancers.

Synthetic progestins, such as Provera, are not found in nature but follow the same hormonal pathways and bind to the same progesterone receptor sites. However, they do not act the same as natural progesterone, and they are not used as precursors for other hormones as is natural progesterone. Provera is the most popular progestin, which is a synthetic compound and is able to maintain the lining of the uterus.

Synthetic progestins can create many unpleasant side effects. They unite with the same receptors as natural progesterone, but carry a different message to the cells. Side effects include fluid retention, breakthrough bleeding, depression, blood clots, acne, hair loss, breast tenderness, jaundice and depression.

The Dangers of Synthetic Hormones

The synthetic progesterone, Provera, has many potential adverse reactions. These include thrombophlebitis and pulmonary embolism. Thrombophlebitis is a blood clot in a vein. A pulmonary embolus is a blood clot in the arterial system to the lung. Other adverse reactions include breakthrough bleeding, spotting, change in menstrual flow, amenorrhea (in which periods completely stop), edema (swelling) and changes in weight (either an increase or decrease). Provera may also cause cholestatic jaundice (a form of yellow jaundice), anaphylactic reactions, rashes, mental depression, insomnia, nausea and prolonged sleepiness.

When synthetic estrogen and progesterones are combined, the adverse reactions may include a rise in blood pressure, PMS, changes in libido, changes in appetite, headaches, nervousness, fatigue, backaches, hirsutism (an increase in body hair), loss of scalp hair, rashes, hemorrhagic eruptions, itching and dizziness.

Natural progesterone may help to protect you

against breast cancer, osteoporosis, endometrial cancer and fibrocystic breast disease. It acts as a natural antidepressant, and it may also improve your sex drive. Many middle-aged women lack this valuable hormone, which may result in an epidemic of anxiety, depression and fatigue. Lack of progesterone may also be setting women up for potentially lethal diseases. Synthetic progesterones have similar protective effects as natural progesterone; however, they may produce many adverse reactions.

Try Nature's Way

Many plants contain estrogen, which is called phytoestrogen. Plant-derived phytoestrogens are found in thousands of different plants. They are primarily extracted from soy beans and tropical wild yams. Diosgenin, a natural progesterone, is usually derived either from soybeans or tropical wild yams. Many products that claim to have wild yam extract may not contain any progesterone. Be sure that you purchase wild yam products containing natural progesterone cream and not the wild yam extract or synthetic progesterone.

Natural progesterone found in phytoestrogens can actually help to alleviate depression. It has a calming effect on the brain.

Natural cream dosage: If you are experiencing premenopausal or menopausal symptoms, I recommend taking natural progesterone cream with approximately 480 milligrams of progesterone per ounce. You can find it at a health food store. Use one-quarter teaspoon of natural progesterone cream twice a day, which is approximately 20 milligrams a day.

Application: Rub this cream on your neck, upper chest, breasts, inner arms, palms and thighs. Rotate the sites. Do not rub it on the same site every day.

Should you take natural progesterone capsules, you must take a much larger dose, since the majority will be excreted almost immediately by the liver if taken orally.

What About Premenopausal Women?

If you are a premenopausal woman, use natural progesterone cream on days twelve through twenty-six of your monthly cycle. (Day one is the first day of your menstrual period.)

Menopausal women may use natural progesterone cream every day of the month. However, if you are taking estrogen hormones, you may need

19

to decrease your amount of estrogen when you begin progesterone, since the progesterone may cause estrogen levels to rise.

Estrogen and progesterone levels may be monitored by blood or saliva testing. I want to reemphasize the fact that you should use natural progesterone

> *You must serve only the LORD your God. If you do, I will bless you with food and water, and I will keep you healthy.*
> —EXODUS 23:25

cream with approximately 480 milligrams of progesterone per ounce, and use only a quarter teaspoon of the cream twice a day. Progesterone creams can be found in all health food stores. However, make sure that it does not contain mineral oil, since mineral oil will prevent the progesterone from being absorbed.

What About Estrogen?

I have talked a lot about progesterone, but what about estrogen? Large numbers of menopausal women in the United States are taking synthetic estrogen and synthetic progesterone to control menopausal symptoms and prevent osteoporosis.

During menopause, estrogen production drops approximately 50 percent. However, progesterone drops significantly more. Many times a woman can raise her estrogen level to normal by simply supplementing with natural progesterone cream. Since natural progesterone is a precursor to estrogen, it can be converted in the body to estrogen. However, if natural progesterone is not controlling the symptoms of menopause, and if the woman is prone to osteoporosis and has a family history of osteoporosis, I recommend that natural estrogen be used as a supplement.

The Problems With Premarin

Horse farms in Canada actually exist for no other reason than to collect the urine from pregnant horses to make the conjugated estrogen tablets called Premarin.

Estrogen patches, which contain 17-beta estradiol, are also popular in the United States. I believe they are safer than the oral synthetic estrogens, which can cause hypertension, fluid retention and blood clots.

Using the Natural Estrogens

The natural estrogen that I prefer to use is triple estrogen or biestrogen. Triple estrogen is 80 percent estriol, 10 percent estradiol and 10 percent estrone. Biestrogen is 90 percent estriol and 10 estradiol. Estriol is the safest form of estrogen with the fewest side effects. Estradiol is a thousand times more potent than estriol in stimulating the breast tissue. Estriol is, therefore, much safer to use than estradiol. You can use triple estrogen in cream form, as in natural progesterone cream, or in capsule form.

If you are menopausal and on estrogen therapy, you should add one-fourth teaspoon of natural progesterone cream applied topically twice a day. Many doctors will tell their patients that since they have had a hysterectomy they do not need progesterone. However, if these women were to have a blood test for progesterone, the level would be extremely low. Therefore, I place all women, whether they have had a hysterectomy or not, on natural progesterone cream or natural progesterone combined with natural estrogen in capsule form. If you cannot find a doctor in your area who prescribes natural progesterone and natural estrogen, I recommend a compounding pharmacy such as Women's International Pharmacy in order to find a physician in your area who prescribes natural hormones. You can contact them at their Web site, www.wipws.com, or at (800) 279-5708.

Control Hot Flashes
With Estriol Creams

By simply using natural progesterone cream, you can usually dramatically decrease your incidence of hot flashes.

Thinning and dryness of the vaginal lining many times is due to the lack of progesterone and estrogen. I recommend that at the onset of hot flashes,

> *Words satisfy the soul as food satisfies the stomach; the right words on a person's lips bring satisfaction.*
> —PROVERBS 18:20

start on natural progesterone cream and use natural estriol cream intravaginally on a daily basis.

Vaginal dryness leads to vaginal itching and burning and thus an increase of vaginal infections. This can also lead to frequent bladder infections. Applying natural estriol cream intravaginally can prevent vaginal and bladder infections. You will need to obtain this cream from a compounding pharmacy such as Women's International Pharmacy, which does require a physician's prescription.

If you are beginning to have symptoms of menopause such as hot flashes and vaginal dryness, consult your physician and have a physical exam. Also obtain a baseline mammogram and a bone density study, the best of which is the Dexa-scan. I would recommend that you not take synthetic estrogens initially, but try the natural progesterone cream and possibly the natural estrogen cream or capsule.

God's Natural Way

God has created a natural pathway for you to walk in divine health. Everything that you need to rise above menopausal symptoms has been provided through natural sources of estrogen and progesterone. You do not have to ingest foreign, synthetic substances into your body to rise above menopause.

You may have been anxious and fearful about going through menopause. At times, you may have experienced symptoms and feelings that were unlike your normal reactions and character. No, you are not changing for the worse. God has created good things for you to rise above menopause. Meditate on His promise:

> For the LORD God is our light and protector. He gives us grace and glory. No good thing will the LORD withhold from those

who do what is right. O LORD Almighty,
happy are those who trust in you.

—PSALM 84:11–12

Thank Him now for the good things—natural progesterone and estrogen sources—that He has created for your health at this important season of transition in your life.

A BIBLE CURE PRAYER
FOR YOU

Lord, I thank You for all the natural options You have created for helping me rise above menopause. Grant me Your wisdom in choosing those natural substances that are best for my body. For every good thing that You have created, I thank You and give You praise. Amen.

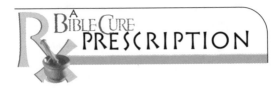

A BIBLE CURE
PRESCRIPTION

Summarize what you have learned about the dangers of synthetic hormone therapy and drugs:

_____

_____

_____

_____

Consult with a physician who understands natural treatments, and write down what that doctor recommends for you about:

Natural progesterone cream: _____

_____

_____

Estriol cream: _____

_____

_____

The effects of synthetic hormones: _____

_____

What choices will you make that will best help you
rise above menopause?

_____

_____

_____

_____

_____

_____

_____

_____

_____

_____

_____

_____

_____

Chapter 3

Embracing Change With Healthy Nutrition

Your health and well-being are very important to God. As a matter of fact, the Bible says that God is always thinking about you!

> How precious are your thoughts about me, O God! They are innumerable! I can't even count them; they outnumber the grains of sand! And when I wake up in the morning, you are still with me!
>
> —Psalm 139:17–18

God's care for you includes providing everything your body needs to function well. He has even given you just the right foods to help you overcome the negative symptoms of menopause. Let's look at the nutrition you need that will help

your body pass through the transition of menopause with comfort and ease.

In the last chapter we examined how phytoestrogens can be applied as creams. Now we can
turn our attention to good nutrition during
menopause, which includes foods that contain
phytoestrogens.

Foods That Contain Estrogen

Did you know that many Asian women who consume high amounts of soy, which is one of the primary phytoestrogens, will rarely have symptoms
of menopause?

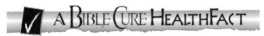

Japanese women have few difficulties and symptoms of menopause. Hot flashes and night sweats
are significantly lower than among Western
women. In a cross-cultural sample with over eight
thousand Massachusetts women and thirteen hundred Canadian women, twelve hundred Japanese
women ages forty-five to fifty-five were compared.
Writing in *Psychosomatic Medicine,* medical
anthropologist Margaret Lock, Ph.D., reported
that these Japanese women have sociological and

biological factors such as diet that lower the symptoms of menopause. Some researchers have suggested that the Asian diet with higher quantities of phytoestrogens lessens the symptoms of menopause.[1]

Foods highest in plant estrogens include:

- Soy
- Flaxseed oil
- Alfalfa
- Fennel seeds
- Flaxseed
- Whole grains
- Parsley
- Celery

Plant-derived estrogens help to balance out the estrogen in your body. If you have high amounts of estrogen, the plant estrogens will lower the estrogens. But if you have low estrogens, the plant estrogens will, by binding to the estrogens, actually raise and balance the estrogen levels. So, phytoestrogens will help to balance your body's estrogen levels.

The Importance of Soy Food Products

The isoflavones in soy are the primary phytoestrogens that your body needs. One cup of soy is equivalent to a regular dose of Premarin. Whole soybean products actually contain higher amounts of isoflavones than other soy protein products. Therefore choose soy flour or whole soy products rather than soy proteins in order to get your phyto-estrogens.

You may also buy capsules of isoflavones or genistein at health food stores to help balance out your estrogen levels.

A BIBLE CURE HEALTH TIP

The Sources of Soy

Don't know tofu from tempeh? Here are some of the most common soy foods, along with a few suggestions for using them.

Meat substitutes—If you want to cut back on meat while getting more soy, look for "mock" meats prepared in the form of cold cuts, bacon, sausage, franks and burgers. These are mainly made from soy, and in some cases they are virtu-ally indistinguishable from the real thing.

Soy flour—Made from roasted, ground soy-beans, soy flour can be used to replace some of the wheat flour used for baking. Nutritionists advise buying defatted soy flour, which contains less fat and more protein that the full-fat variety.

Soy milk—A creamy, milk-like drink made

from ground, soaked soybeans and water, it's sold plain and in a variety of flavors. Some people prefer "lite" soy milk. It's lower fat than the regular kind, but it may contain fewer of the protective phytoestrogens.

Tempeh—These chunky, tender cakes are made from fermented soybeans that have been laced with mold, giving them their distinctive smoky, nutty flavor. You can grill tempeh or add it to spaghetti sauce, chili or casseroles.

Texturized soy protein—Made from soy flour, this meat substitute can replace part or all of the meat in meatloaf, burgers and chili.

<u>**Tofu**</u>—A creamy white, soft, cheeselike food made from curdled soy milk. Tofu comes in firm and soft varieties and can be used in virtually anything from soups to desserts. You will find soft and firm varieties of tofu at most supermarkets in the produce section. Other soy foods are available at specialty and health food stores.[2]

Phytoestrogens also block out estradiol and toxic xenoestrogens. Xenoestrogens are chemicals such as petroleum-based products that have estrogen-like activity. Phytoestrogens will help your body decrease hot flashes, prevent osteoporosis and assist your body in preventing vaginal dryness. In addition, diets that are high in phytoestrogens protect against breast and colon cancers.

Two Diets to Avoid

The two main hormones made by the ovaries—estrogen and progesterone—are two of the steroid hormones in the body. Steroid hormones actu-

> *But those who wait on the LORD will find new strength. They will fly high on wings like eagles. They will run and not grow weary. They will walk and not faint.*
> —ISAIAH 40:31

ally come from cholesterol, and most of the steroid hormones are very similar in shape. However, they have extremely different effects. The steroid hormones include progesterone, estrogen, pregnenolone, DHEA, androstenedione, testosterone, cortisol, aldosterone and others.

Since all of these steroid hormones are made from cholesterol, it is critically important never to go on a no-cholesterol or a no-fat diet. If you eliminate all cholesterol foods and fats from your diet, you may develop a hormone imbalance since all of the steroid hormones come from cholesterol.

Choosing the Oils in Your Diet

Oils to avoid

Hydrogenated oils and partially hydrogenated oils are probably the most dangerous oils that you can consume. If you are a menopausal or pre-menopausal woman, avoid or decrease hydrogenated oils and most heat-processed vegetable oils in your diet. Hydrogenated oils and partially hydrogenated oils are man-made oils such as margarine. They are found in potato chips, most baked goods, candies and most processed foods. Unsaturated vegetable oils such as corn oil, safflower oil, sunflower oil and peanut oil have been heat processed and are very unstable and nearly always turn rancid. Rancid oil causes oxidation in the body, which leads to degenerative diseases such as heart disease and cancer.

Margarines are actually vegetable oils heated to very high temperatures under high pressure, which transforms them into unnatural hardened oils. A small amount of organic butter on occasion is much healthier than eating hydrogenated fats or heat-processed unsaturated vegetable oils. Cold-processed unsaturated vegetable oils found in health food stores are much healthier. Olestra is a fat substitute found in many snack foods such as potato chips. It can limit the absorption of carotenoids, which are rich yellow, orange and red vegetables as well as dark green leafy vegetables, by as much as 50 percent.

Polyunsaturated fats and saturated fats actually form our cell membranes. However, our bodies do not know what to do with the hydrogenated fats such as margarine. Since they are foreign to our bodies, they have a harmful effect on our cell membranes, our blood vessels and our immune systems. Thus they may significantly increase your risk of developing heart disease or cancer.

Unsaturated vegetable oils that are heat processed, such as corn oil, safflower oil, sunflower oil and peanut oil, cause oxidation in the body, which may damage tissues. Excessive amounts of these oils lead to an imbalance in female hormones.

Oils that are good for you

Olive and fish oils—One of the best oils to use is extra-virgin olive oil. Fish oil in capsule form or from eating fatty fish such as salmon, mackerel, herring, halibut and tuna is a good source of essential fats.

Flaxseed oil—I recommend taking one

tablespoon of flaxseed oil daily. However, keep it refrigerated. Do not cook with this oil because it is easily damaged by heat and light. Flaxseed oil is one of the most important oils to be consumed by menopausal women. High lignan flaxseed oil is high in plant estrogens. Foods high in plant estrogens such as soy and flaxseed oil will help balance out the estrogen, thus helping to control menopausal symptoms.

One of the highest-quality flaxseed oils is Barlean's Flax Oil. This oil is extracted at temperatures below 96 degrees, which protects the oil from rancidity caused by heat, oxygen and light. Flaxseed oil contains the essential

> *Those who have been ransomed by the LORD will return to Jerusalem, singing songs of everlasting joy. Sorrow and mourning will disappear, and they will be overcome with joy and gladness.*
> —ISAIAH 51:11

fatty acids alpha-linolenic and lenoleic. It also contains high amounts of Omega-3 fatty acids, which have beneficial effects in preventing heart disease, arthritis and allergic disorders.

I personally take a tablespoon of flaxseed oil twice a day. You may add it to salad dressings or to foods after they have been cooked. Ground flaxseed, in addition to flaxseed oil, is high in the fiber lignin, which has cancer-fighting properties. Lignin in flaxseed reduces estrogen by preventing it from being recirculated through the liver. Thus it is able to help relieve hot flashes. Grind five teaspoons of organic flaxseed in a coffee grinder and blend it with your favorite soy/protein drink each morning.

Junk Food and You

Often women who experience symptoms caused by menopause and premenopause do not turn to eating healthy food, but instead they start consuming junk foods and high-sugar foods, including cakes, pies, cookies and starchy foods like breads, pasta, potatoes and chips. They also consume stimulants such as caffeine, which is contained in coffee, cola, tea and chocolate. Unfortunately, many women even turn to alcohol and prescription drugs in order to relieve their stress.

As a result, many women don't get the essential vitamins and minerals and the overall nutrition that they need to maintain an adequate hormonal balance. Because of this lack of nutrition, women can begin having menstrual cycles in which they do not ovulate—even as early as a decade prior to the onset of menopause.

You can balance your hormones and thus delay or lessen the symptoms of premenopause by learning to avoid the following:

- Junk foods
- Processed foods
- Alcohol
- Margarine
- Sugar
- Caffeine
- Fried foods

Instead, learn to select foods that are nutritionally healthy for you. Choose:

- Fresh fruits
- Lean meats
- Fresh vegetables
- Whole grains
- "Good" fats that your body needs (seeds, nuts, olive oil and avocado)
- A comprehensive multivitamin/multimineral tablet

Nutritional Steps

Limit red meat. Do not overindulge in red meats. Many of our cattle are injected with estrogens to increase their weight. The estrogen is concentrated in the fatty tissues, and when you eat the meat, the estrogens in the meat will accumulate in your body.

Instead of choosing red meat and pork, eat more fish—especially the fatty fish such as salmon, mackerel, herring, halibut and tuna. In addition, eat more fiber since it will unite with estrogen in the GI tract and prevent it from being reabsorbed back into the blood stream.

Avoid high-fat dairy products. Menopausal women should decrease or avoid high-fat dairy products such as whole milk, whole milk cheeses and butter. Instead, you should choose skim milk and skim milk cheeses. Also avoid fatty meats since both high-fat dairy products and fatty meats can promote

> *Praise the LORD, I tell myself; with my whole heart, I will praise his holy name. Praise the LORD, I tell myself, and never forget the good things he does for me. He forgives all my sins and heals all my diseases.*
> —PSALM 103:1–3

hot flashes. It is best to eat unprocessed, whole-grain foods, fruits and vegetables. Processed foods can constipate the body and lead to more menopausal and premenopausal symptoms.

Eat fresh vegetables. Fresh vegetables eaten raw, steamed or stir-fried cleanse the body and prevent many menopausal symptoms. Choose organic vegetables and fruits over regular supermarket fruits and vegetables. Pesticides sprayed on supermarket fruits and vegetables can lead to the development of estrogen dominance and pre-menopausal symptoms as early as a decade or two before menopause occurs.

Eat Superfoods

Other sources of phytoestrogens include alfalfa, parsley and celery, which have higher amounts of phytoestrogens. Eat these superfood vegetables for their strong antioxidant properties and phytonutrients that protect from heart disease and cancer.

The strong antioxidant function of these superfoods will help your body to resist degenerative diseases. Superfoods also help you to maintain a proper hormonal balance.

Eat your carotenoids. Carotenoids are usually orange foods, but may also include dark green vegetables. They include carrots, watermelons, tomatoes, cantaloupe, pink grapefruit, sweet potatoes, squash and spinach. Carotenoids may lower the risk of developing cancer and are very important in immune function.

Include lycopene-rich foods in your menus. The next group of superfoods are the lycopene-rich foods, which are the red foods. Lycopene is found in tomatoes, carrots, pink grapefruit, watermelon, apricots and strawberries. High consumption of lycopene foods will reduce the risk of prostate cancer and heart attacks.

You need cruciferous vegetables. Cruciferous vegetables are the next group of superfoods. These include broccoli, cauliflower, cabbage, Brussels sprouts and kale. They have potent phytonutrients that are important in helping to prevent breast cancer.

Eat grass—really! Green superfoods are high in chlorophyll. These include spirulina, chlorella, blue-green algae, barley grass, wheat grass and alfalfa. These vegetables contain almost every mineral and trace mineral necessary for human survival. They also cleanse our bodies of toxins and poisons and protect them from the damaging affects of these toxins.

Consume fruit. Citrus fruits such as oranges, lemons and grapefruit are high in vitamin C. Vitamin C has antioxidant activity and works synergistically to help recycle vitamin E. Vitamin C is also found in berries and green vegetables such as asparagus, broccoli, spinach, turnip greens and dandelion greens.

Drink lots of water. I strongly recommend that women drink one and one-half to two quarts of filtered or distilled water a day. It helps to rid the body of toxins and will help keep the colon and digestive tracts functioning normally.

Stay away from fast foods. Often menopausal symptoms begin ten to fifteen years before menopause actually begins. Today's woman faces many high-stress demands: working a job, raising a family, shopping and cleaning. When combined with poor diets of fast foods, very few fruits and vegetables, high-sugar intake, processed foods with low fiber, in addition to exposure to pesticides, herbicides and xenoestrogens from fatty meats, cheese, whole milk and ice cream, it leads eventually to non-ovulating menstrual cycles.

Hidden Chemicals

Xenoestrogens are environmental chemicals that are usually petrochemical by-products from plastics, solvents, herbicides and pesticides. Many of these compounds have very high estrogenic activity, and they are fat-soluble and nonbiodegradable. These chemical estrogens are actually much more potent than estrogens made by the ovaries. I believe this is one of the main reasons why we are seeing such an epidemic of breast cancer and other female cancers in the industrialized world.

These xenoestrogens are unknowingly consumed in our diets. No one in their right mind would consume pesticides, herbicides, petrochemicals, solvents or plastic materials. However, animals, especially cows and pigs, accumulate these pesticides, herbicides and petrochemicals in their fatty tissues. Pesticides are sprayed on the grains the animals eat, and then the poisons are concentrated in their fatty tissues.

These animals are also given estrogenic compounds in order to gain more weight. When you eat a fatty, greasy hamburger or bacon, cheese or ice cream, or when you drink whole milk, you are getting a relatively high amount

> *May God our Father and the Lord Jesus Christ give you his grace and peace. I can never stop thanking God for all the generous gifts he has given you, now that you belong to Christ Jesus.*
> —1 CORINTHIANS 1:3–4

of pesticides that are concentrated in these animal fats. These pesticides will collect in your own fatty tissues, including the breasts and the brain. They can also bind to the estrogen receptor and may stimulate the receptor, thus forming more estrogen, or block the receptor, thus blocking the normal function of the estrogen.

Watch Out for Environmental Toxins

I believe that excessive estrogen stimulation by these xenoestrogens is a factor in the development of breast cancer and other cancers. I have lived in the greater Orlando, Florida, area for the past sixteen years. In the Orlando suburb of Apopka, there is a very large lake called Lake Apopka. In 1980 there was a pesticide spill in Lake Apopka. Since then, the number of young alligators in that lake has decreased. Be on the alert for toxins in your environment.

Listening to God

God can help you choose what to eat while overcoming the temptation to eat foods harmful to your body. He wants you to prosper and be in good health. Not only does proper nutrition help you rise above the negative symptoms of menopause, it also strengthens your immune system so that you can prevent and fight off any attacks of disease.

Before you go shopping, ask God to guide you in preparing a shopping list to help you buy the right foods. Before ordering a meal in a restaurant, ask the Lord to help you select foods on the menu that are best for you. The Bible promises that you can do all things through Him who strengthens you (Phil. 4:13).

You are not condemned to live with menopausal pain and discomfort. You are not a victim of life's changes. You are a victor over everything in life. So rise above your physical circumstances and develop self-control over what you eat. God gives you self-control so that you can walk in divine health and be physically able to serve Him at home, work, church and in every situation of life.

A BIBLE CURE PRAYER FOR YOU

Spirit of God, help me to make right choices when I shop for food or order a meal in a restaurant. Strengthen my resolve to eat right so that I may rise above menopause and live a healthy, pain-free life. Lord, Your wisdom can guide my every decision so that I will take care of this temple, my body, which is a gift from You. Thank You for creating all the right foods I need in order to eat wholesome foods that lessen and prevent the symptoms of menopause. Thank You, Lord. Amen.

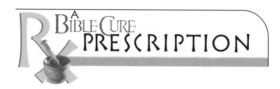

Toward a Healthy Nutritional Lifestyle

List the five types of foods you will avoid eating in order to help your body rise above menopause:

_____

_____

List at least five healthy choices of foods you will make this week as you plan your menus:

_____

_____

Write a prayer asking God to help you make right nutritional choices.

_____

_____

_____

_____

Chapter 4

Embracing
Change With Vitamins
and Supplements

Y our body is extremely important in God's
eyes—in fact, the Bible says it is the temple of
God's Spirit. First Corinthians 3:16 says:

> Don't you realize that all of you together
> are the temple of God and that the Spirit of
> God lives in you?

God created ways for you to use natural substances to help you feel better during this season
of transition. Taking certain vitamins and supplements will greatly reduce any of the adverse
symptoms of menopause. The following list of
vitamins and supplements will enable you to rise
above menopause.

Vitamin E taken internally at a dosage of 800

international units daily may help menopausal symptoms. Vitamin E cream applied to the vaginal area may prevent itching.

Vitamin C with bioflavonoids such as hesperidin and quercetin may help relieve hot flashes. Take at least 1,000 milligrams daily of both vitamin C and bioflavonoids.

✓ **Lecithin granules** in a dose of 1 tablespoon two to three times a day before meals may also help to reduce hot flashes.

Evening primrose oil, borage oil and black currant seed oil may also relieve hot flashes, as well as gamma-oryzanol, which is a component of rice bran oil. Take approximately 300 milligrams a day of gamma-oryzanol. You should take enough evening primrose, borage or black currant oil to equal 300 milligrams of the fatty acid GLA a day.

A multivitamin/multimineral supplement is recommended for menopausal women.

Calcium should be taken in a dose of 1,500 milligrams a day with 400 units of vitamin D.

Magnesium and boron should be taken in a dose of 400 milligrams of magnesium and 3 milligrams of boron a day. This will help to prevent osteoporosis.

Herbs That Can Help

Herbs may also be helpful in controlling menopausal symptoms. Try the following:

Black cohosh comes from a shrub that is native to the forests of North America. Its black root is one of the main constituents used in the herbal preparation. The word *cohosh* is an Indian word that means "rough." Native American Indians used this herb for many different problems, including menopausal symptoms, menstrual cramps and even rattlesnake bites.

During menopause, estrogen production usually slows down and another hormone, called LH or the luteinizing hormone, increases. As a result of the increasing LH and decreasing estrogen, hot flashes occur. Black cohosh has weak estrogen-like activity, and it may decrease the LH secretion, thus reducing hot flashes. I recommend the standardized extract of the herb, which contains 1 milligram per tablet.

> *To all who mourn in Israel, he will give beauty for ashes, joy instead of mourning, praise instead of despair. For the LORD has planted them like strong and graceful oaks for his own glory.*
> —ISAIAH 61:3

An excellent product that contains black cohosh is Remifemin.

Dong quai is a plant that is a member of the celery family. It is often referred to in Chinese medicine as female ginseng. It tends to help balance the feminine hormonal system. Dong quai is not a phytoestrogen like soy and does not exhibit any hormone-like actions in the body. Dong quai relieves hot flashes during the perimenopausal period. By balancing female hormones, it relieves painful menstruation or too frequent menstruation.

The root of the plant is used for medicinal purposes. The powdered root can be purchased at a health food store in capsule, tablet or tea forms. A common dose of dong quai capsules is 1 to 2 grams, three times a day.

Chasteberry, also called *vitex,* has been used since ancient times to suppress libido and inspire chastity. The whole-fruit extract of the chasteberry is used. The chasteberry contains no hormones. However, it is believed to be able to increase production of progesterone, thus helping to regulate a woman's menstrual cycle.

Chasteberry does not work rapidly. It usually takes months for this hormone to start balancing the woman's hormonal system. Powdered extracts are usually taken in a dose of 250 to 500 milligrams three times a day.

Licorice root has been used for thousands of years in China. Licorice not only relieves PMS, but it may also lower estrogen while raising progesterone levels. In doing so, it may relieve many symptoms of menopause. The two main components of licorice are flavonoids and glycyrrhiza. Glycyrrhiza may cause an increase in blood pressure and water retention, so people with hypertension or edema should avoid this product. The normal dose of licorice is 250 to 500 milligrams three times a day. Have your blood pressure checked periodically while on this supplement.

Ginkgo biloba should normally be taken in a dose of approximately 40 milligrams, one to two tablets, two to three times a day. Make sure that it is the standardized extract of 24 percent flavone glycosides.

Genistein is the main isoflavone found in soy. Isoflavone is the main plant estrogen and can be obtained in powder, capsule or tablet form. Genistein may be taken in pill or capsule form, approximately 50 milligrams a day. You can find this at a health food store.

What About Promensil?

Another natural phytoestrogen product available to you is Promensil. Promensil is a soy supplement that contains 40 milligrams of isoflavones per tablet. There are many different soy extracts that contain similar amounts of isoflavones. Isoflavones are phytoestrogens that are found in soy.

In Japan, soy is consumed in much greater quantities than here in the United States. As a result, Japanese men and women have approximately one-fourth the rates of breast and prostate cancer as do American men and women. The typical daily intake of isoflavones in Japan is estimated to be around 50 milligrams per day per person. In the United States it is estimated that the typical daily intake is only 2 or 3 milligrams a day.

✓ A BIBLE CURE HEALTHFACT

Did you know that there isn't even a word in Japanese for "hot flash?"

Consider this: In Asian countries where women eat a lot of soy foods, only 16 percent of women have a problem with menopausal discomfort. In this country, however, where soy foods are used much less often, 75 percent of menopausal

women complain of hot flashes or other uncomfortable symptoms.[1]

Soy Extracts

You can purchase many soy extracts in capsule form that provide high levels of isoflavones. Two capsules of megasoy extract contain 100 milligrams of isoflavones. It is best to take one capsule twice a day. However, women who do not wish to take estrogen may take two to three capsules of soy extract such as megasoy extract or Promensil, or another type of soy extract that contains about 50 milligrams of isoflavone per capsule, twice a day.

> *Don't worry about anything; instead, pray about everything. Tell God what you need, and thank him for all he has done. If you do this, you will experience God's peace, which is far more wonderful than the human mind can understand. His peace will guard your hearts and minds as you live in Christ Jesus.*
> —PHILIPPIANS 4:6–7

This may prove to be an adequate estrogen replacement therapy for many women. However, you should consult your physician to make sure

53

that your estrogen level is adequate enough to prevent osteoporosis.

A Final Note

As you make choices concerning your supplements and vitamins, consult a nutritional doctor and spend time in prayer and the Scriptures seeking God's guidance. There are many wonderful substances to help your body overcome the uncomfortable symptoms of menopause and to prevent any physical attacks on your body.

Not only are you seeking to rise above menopause, you are taking care of your body, which is the temple of God's Spirit. When you take care of yourself, you will be available to God to serve Him and others in love.

A BIBLE CURE PRAYER
FOR YOU

O God, fill me with the wisdom, commitment and determination to take care of my temple so that I may serve and glorify You in all that I do. I want to live a long, prosperous and healthy life in order to serve and honor You in all ways. Thank You for the knowledge of vitamins and supplements that help to strengthen my immune system and to overcome any adverse symptoms of menopause. Amen.

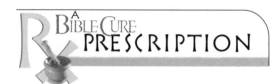

A BIBLE CURE PRESCRIPTION

Check the following vitamins and supplements you (along with the advice of your doctor and/or nutritionist) have determined that you need.

- ❏ Vitamin E (800 I.U. daily)
- ❏ Vitamin C and bioflavonoids (1,000 mg. daily)
- ❏ Lecithin granules (1–2 tbsp., 2–3 times daily before meals)
- ❏ Evening primrose oil, borage oil or black currant seed oil (equal to 300 mg. of GLA)
- ❏ A good multivitamin and multimineral
- ❏ Calcium (1,500 mg. daily)
- ❏ Vitamin D (400 I.U. daily)
- ❏ Magnesium (400 mg. daily)
- ❏ Boron (3 mg. daily)
- ❏ Black cohosh (1 mg. tablet daily)
- ❏ Dong quai (1–2 gram tablet, 3 times daily)
- ❏ Chasteberry (250–500 mg. tablet, 3 times daily)
- ❏ Licorice root (250–500 mg. tablets, 3 times daily)
- ❏ Ginkgo biloba (40 mg. tablet, 2–3 times daily)
- ❏ Genistein (50 mg. daily)
- ❏ Promensil (check with your physician)

Chapter 5

Embracing Change With Exercise and Weight Loss

The most beautiful season of the year is autumn. But too many women think of the autumn season of their lives as a time of loss: losing one's youth, one's figure, one's energy and stamina. You may choose to look at your new season as such—but you don't have to. The choice is yours!

I believe our Creator had a reason for making autumn so beautiful. The autumn of your life can be just as beautiful. But you must boldly embrace this season and make it all that it can be. I know you'll be pleasantly surprised if you do. You will be the most beautiful person you've ever been in the autumn of your life. Remember God's promise: "He has made everything beautiful in its time" (Eccles. 3:11, NKJV). So, embrace this autumn season of your life. It is your time, and God has made you beautiful in it!

One way to embrace this time of life is to make it all it can be through determined effort. Your body will respond to your control as you master it. The apostle Paul understood this mind-set. Look at what he said:

> Remember that in a race everyone runs, but only one person gets the prize. You also must run in such a way that you will win. All athletes practice strict self-control. They do it to win a prize that will fade away, but we do it for an eternal prize. So I run straight to the goal with purpose in every step. I am not like a boxer who misses his punches. I discipline my body like an athlete, training it to do what it should. Otherwise, I fear that after preaching to others I myself might be disqualified.
>
> —1 CORINTHIANS 9:24–27

Paul wasn't one of the greatest apostles by accident. He made up his mind, and God helped him to be all that he could be. God will help you, too!

Your body needs to be maintained in divine health through weight loss and exercise. Obesity is a major cause of estrogen dominance, which leads to premenopausal symptoms. As you recall, fatty tissue will cause an increased production of estrogen.

Do You Love to Walk?

I recommend taking a twenty- to thirty-minute brisk walk every other day. Or find another exercise that you enjoy and can do at least three to four times a week. Regular exercise can make all the difference during this season of your life. It helps keep your metabolism high, which prevents weight gain, and it reduces the effects and intensity of hot flashes.

Exercising and maintaining a healthy diet are difficult to do alone. I recommend that you find another woman who has successfully gone through menopause as your prayer and exercise partner. You can support one another in your commitment to exercise and eat right.

A Walking Program

Here's a walking program to help get you exercising. Don't look at walking as work. Instead, choose to see it as "your time," a special time for you to get away and enjoy the outdoors, fresh air and the wonders of God's creation.

Always get a checkup before starting an exercise program. Begin walking at a pace that is comfortable for you. However, you should walk briskly enough so that you cannot sing, but not so briskly that you cannot talk.

A BIBLE CURE HEALTH TIP

A Simple Walking Program

(NOTE: Each column indicates the number of minutes to walk. Complete three exercise sessions each week. If you find a particular week's pattern tiring, repeat it before going on to the next pattern. You do not have to complete the walking program in twelve weeks.)

Week	—Walk	—Walk Briskly	—Walk	—Minutes
1	5	5	5	15
2	5	7	5	17
3	5	9	5	19
4	5	11	5	21
5	5	13	5	23
6	5	15	5	25
7	5	18	5	28
8	5	20	5	30

9	5	23	5	33
10	5	26	5	36
11	5	28	5	38
12	5	30	5	40

Week 13 and thereafter: Check your pulse periodically to see if you are exercising within your target zone. As you get more in shape, try exercising within the upper range of your target zone. Gradually increase your brisk walking time from 30 to 60 minutes, three or four times a week. Remember that your goal is to get the benefits you are seeking and enjoy your activity.

You can obtain a heart rate monitor that straps around your chest to calculate your heart rate while you walk.

Your Predicted Heart Rate

Use the following chart to determine your target heart rate while exercising. Once you have determined your desired heart rate range, write down your actual heart rate after each walking session or other exercise.

Calculate your target heart zone using this formula:

220 minus [your age] = _____
x .65 = _____
[This is your minimum.]
220 minus [your age] = _____
x .80 = _____
[This is your maximum.]

This example may help: To calculate the target heart zone for a 40-year-old man, subtract the age (40) from 220 (220- 40=180). Multiply 180 by .65, which equals 117. Then multiply 180 by .80, which equals 144. A 40-year-old man's target heart rate zone is 117–144 beats per minute.

Hanging In There

You may be thinking, *I've tried many exercise programs, but I never hang in there long enough to get results. I always quit too soon.* Here's a tip: Make your walking program a vital part of your day. Too many people get into trouble when they save exercising for their spare time. If you wait until you can get around to it, you probably never will.

Choose an exercise activity that you truly enjoy.

Walking is only one suggestion. Have you tried bicycling? Or golfing (without a golfcart)? Perhaps you've always pictured yourself on a tennis court.

Aerobic exercise such as brisk walking, swimming and cycling will also help to dissipate the stress, thus delaying the symptoms of pre-menopause.

Recharge your body every night by getting at least seven to eight hours of good, restful sleep. This will not only recharge your body, but also your mind. It will help prevent irritability, anxiety, depression and fatigue.

Remember, this is *your* special season. Do this for you! Each day as you start out, ask God for the determination to hang in there. You'll be surprised at the results.

Most people feel calm and have a sense of well-being after they

> *Spend your time and energy in training yourself for fitness. Physical exercise has some value, but spiritual exercise is much more important, for it promises a reward in both this life and the next.*
> —1 TIMOTHY 4:7–8

exercise. You can actually walk off your anxieties. People who exercise feel better about themselves, look better, feel more energetic and are more productive at work.

A BIBLE CURE PRAYER
FOR YOU

Lord, help me make and maintain good eating and exercise habits. Thank You for the temple of my body. Give me the desire and determination to follow Your directions in caring for the gift of my body. Amen.

What Would You Like to Weigh?

Suppose you could wake up tomorrow morning with the body weight that is perfect for you. What would that be? You may have given up on enjoying your ideal body weight a long time ago. You shouldn't have. Now is the best time for you to enjoy your life! So, set a goal.

Following is a chart of your goal weight. Find your height and frame size and write down your goal weight in the space provided.

My goal weight is ____ pounds.
My actual weight is ____ pounds.
I need to lose ___ pounds.

Height and Weight Table for Women

Height	Small Frame	Medium Frame	Large Frame
4'10"	102–111 lbs.	109–121 lbs.	118–131 lbs.
4'11"	103–113 lbs.	111–123 lbs.	120–134 lbs.
5'0"	104–115 lbs.	113–126 lbs.	122–137 lbs.
5'1"	106–118 lbs.	115–129 lbs.	125–140 lbs.
5'2"	108–121 lbs.	118–132 lbs.	128–143 lbs.
5'3"	111–124 lbs.	121–135 lbs.	131–147 lbs.
5'4"	114–127 lbs.	124–138 lbs.	134–151 lbs.
5'5"	117–130 lbs.	127–141 lbs.	137–155 lbs.
5'6"	120–133 lbs.	130–144 lbs.	140–159 lbs.
5'7"	123–136 lbs.	133–147 lbs.	143–163 lbs.
5'8"	126–139 lbs.	136–150 lbs.	146–167 lbs.
5'9"	129–142 lbs.	139–153 lbs.	149–170 lbs.
5'10"	132–145 lbs.	142–156 lbs.	152–173 lbs.
5'11"	135–148 lbs.	145–159 lbs.	155–176 lbs.
6'0"	138–151 lbs.	148–162 lbs.	158–179 lbs.

Nothing Is Impossible!

Feel like you'll never be at your ideal weight? Don't be discouraged. The Bible says that with faith, nothing is impossible. Look at this powerful scripture:

> I assure you, even if you had faith as small as a mustard seed you could say to this mountain, "Move from here to there," and it would move. Nothing would be impossible.
>
> —MATTHEW 17:20

Faith is the most powerful force in the universe. A person with a little faith can conquer every foe—even those extra pounds that have been defeating you for so long! Faith is not an emotion. It's not an eerie force. Faith is a decision to choose to believe God no matter what you see or feel. Faith is so simple!

Make the choice right now to believe that God can help you to overcome anything in your life that is defeating you. Give Him all of your challenges. I promise that you won't be sorry.

A BIBLE CURE PRAYER
FOR YOU

Lord Jesus, I choose to believe that the power of the cross is greater than my bondage to obesity. You love me and died on the cross to free me from all of my bondages. I, (your name), choose faith today (date). I give You these (how many pounds) pounds—my mountain of obesity. In Jesus' name, I declare victory today! Amen.

Daily Weight Loss Steps

This Bible cure plan combines faith in God with practical steps, as you know by now. So, here is the practical side: the diet. God urges you not to eat animal fats—one of the main contributors to weight gain. He commands, "You must never eat any fat or blood. This is a permanent law for you and all your descendants, wherever they may live" (Lev. 3:17).

Although we are no longer under the ancient Hebrew dietary laws, the principles of healthy nutrition remain timeless.

I recommend you use the rules of good nutrition and create a daily diet using these menu planning tips.

A BIBLE CURE HEALTH TIP

Sample Menu	*Improved Higher Fiber Menu*
BREAKFAST	**BREAKFAST**
$\frac{1}{2}$ c. orange juice	$\frac{1}{2}$ c. orange juice
1 piece whole-grain toast	1 oz. Fiber One
1 tbsp. cream cheese	$\frac{1}{2}$ cup berries
1 c. skim milk	1 c. skim milk
LUNCH	**LUNCH**
2 oz. chicken salad on	2 oz. chicken salad on
2 slices whole-grain bread	2 slices whole-wheat bread
$\frac{1}{2}$ c. carrot sticks	1 small apple
1 glass green tea with Stevia	$\frac{1}{2}$ c. carrot sticks
	1 glass green tea with Stevia
DINNER	**DINNER**
3 oz. grilled salmon	3 oz. grilled salmon
$\frac{1}{2}$ c. broccoli	$\frac{1}{2}$ c. broccoli
1 whole-grain roll	1 serving brown rice
1 tsp. butter or Smart Balance	2 tsp. butter or Smart Balance
$\frac{1}{2}$ c. strawberries	$\frac{1}{2}$ c. strawberries
1 c. head lettuce with	1 c. Romaine lettuce with
2 tbsp. French dressing	2 tbsp. French dressing
1 c. skim milk	1 c. skim milk
SNACKS	**SNACKS**
6 oz. yogurt	2 c. melon
1 apple	1 apple

Simple Rules

The following are simple dieting rules I recommend to my patients who need to lose weight.

1. Graze throughout the day. (Eat lots of salads and veggies often throughout the day.)
2. Eat a fairly large breakfast.
3. Eat smaller midmorning, mid-afternoon and evening snacks.
4. Avoid all simple sugar foods such as candies, cookies, cakes, pies and doughnuts. If you must have sugar, use either Stevia or Sweet Balance (found in health food stores).
5. Drink 2 quarts of filtered or bottled water a day. It is best to drink two 8-ounce glasses 30 minutes before each meal, or one to two 8-ounce glasses 2½ hours after each meal.
6. Avoid alcohol.
7. Avoid all fried foods and decrease intake of animal fats (whole milk, cheese, fatty cuts of meat, bacon, sausage, ham, etc.).
8. Avoid, or decrease dramatically, starches. Starches include all breads,

crackers, bagels, potatoes, pasta, rice, corn, black beans, pinto beans and red beans. Also limit your intake of bananas.

9. Eat fresh fruits; steamed, stir-fried or raw vegetables; lean meats; salads (preferably with extra-virgin olive oil and vinegar); nuts (almonds, organic peanuts) and seeds.

10. Take fiber supplements such as Fiber Plus, Perdiem Fiber or any other fiber without NutraSweet or sugar.

11. Take 2 tablespoons of milk of magnesia each day if constipated. However, first make sure you are consuming at least 35 grams of fiber each day and drinking 2–3 quarts of water a day.

12. For snacks, choose Iron Man PR Bars, Zone Bars or Balance Bars. My favorite snack bar is the yogurt honey peanut Balance Bars. These may be purchased at a health food store.

13. Do not eat past 7 P.M.

So, Get Started

With God on your side, you will win! Psalm 56:9 says, "This I know: God is on my side." All the help you need to have victory with weight loss and exercise is just a prayer away! So, make a bold commitment right now to get started today.

A BIBLE CURE PRAYER FOR YOU

Lord, I surrender the entire issue of weight control to You. Help me to face this issue in my life and find new hope, fresh vision and powerful victory in You. Your Word says, "Nothing is impossible with God." I choose to believe Your Word right now above my feelings of defeat in the arena of weight control. Thank You for loving me just as I am. And thank You for helping me to control my weight so that I will live a longer and better life. Amen.

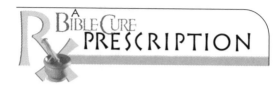

A BIBLE CURE PRESCRIPTION

Write out a menu for the coming week to start your weight loss program:

_____

_____

_____

_____

_____

_____

_____

_____

Describe the exercise you are getting daily now:

_____

_____

_____

_____

How are you monitoring your heart rate?

_____

_____

_____

_____

_____

_____

What exercise will you commit yourself to start in
the coming week?

_____

_____

_____

_____

_____

_____

_____

_____

_____

Chapter 6

Embracing Faith in Seasons of Change

Have you experienced concerns over your symptoms of menopause and doubts about yourself when you feel out of sorts? Rest assured that nothing about your life has gone out of control. God is gracing your life with a wonderful season of change. This special time of change is from Him. The Bible says, "And He changes the times and the seasons" (Dan. 2:21, NKJV).

Embrace your new season with grace, excitement and peace through the power of faith. The Bible says, "You will keep in perfect peace all who trust in you, whose thoughts are fixed on you!" (Isa. 26:3).

You can strengthen your faith through the Word of God. The Bible says, "So then faith comes by hearing, and hearing by the word of God"

(Rom. 10:17, NKJV). Reading the Bible, meditating upon the many scripture verses throughout this booklet and praying often will strengthen your faith and help you to transition from this season to the next with grace and peace.

Overcoming Stress With Faith

Stress can be a big factor during menopause and premenopause. American women are entering this season of life at an early age. I believe that it is due to the tremendous stress of their lifestyles. The hormonal balance of estrogen and progesterone, as well as deficiencies of these hormones, relates to the amount of stress you may be facing daily.

You can take Bible Cure steps immediately to reduce your stress. Follow these simple, spiritual steps:

Fix your attention on Jesus—not on your problems.

Dwelling on your problems produces inner turmoil and blocks the power of Christ, the Prince of Peace, from comforting and calming you. Follow this Bible Cure prescription: "Therefore, since we are surrounded by such a huge crowd of witnesses to the life of faith, let us strip off every weight that slows us down, especially the sin that so easily hinders our progress. And let us run with endurance the race that God has set before us. We do this by keeping our eyes on Jesus, on whom our faith depends from start to finish. He was willing to die a shameful death on the cross because of the joy he knew would be his afterward. Now he is seated in the place of highest honor beside God's throne in heaven" (Heb. 12:1–2).

Pray and thank God for all His blessings.

> *For God has not given us a spirit of fear and timidity, but of power, love, and self-discipline.*
> —2 TIMOTHY 1:7

When stressed, you may tend to forget all that God has done and is doing in your life. Your blessings far outweigh any temporary crisis. As you pray for your needs, also thank God for His providential care: "So I tell you, don't worry about everyday life—whether you have enough food, drink, and clothes. Doesn't life consist of more than food and clothing? Look at the birds. They don't need to plant or harvest or put food in barns because your heavenly Father feeds them. And you are far more valuable to him than they are" (Matt. 6:25–26).

Eliminate negative thoughts by meditating on uplifting thoughts.

Scripture reveals that you become what you think (Prov. 23:7, NKJV). Instead of dwelling on what stresses you, clean out negative thoughts, replacing them with the joy-filled attitudes described in the Bible: "Always be full of joy in the Lord. I say it again—rejoice! . . . Don't worry about anything; instead, pray about everything. Tell God what you need, and thank him for all he has done. If you do this, you will experience God's peace, which is far more wonderful than the human mind can understand. His peace will guard your hearts and minds as you live in Christ Jesus. And now, dear friends, let me say one more thing as I close this letter. Fix your thoughts on what is true and honorable and right. Think about things that are pure and lovely and admirable. Think about things that are excellent and worthy of praise" (Phil. 4:4, 6–8).

Take the One-Year-to-Live Test

Take the "one-year-to-live-test." Pretend that you have only one year to live. What would you do during that time? Divide the things you would do into three categories:

1. Things you enjoy doing
2. Activities you must do
3. Activities you neither enjoy nor have to do

Now, eliminate all activities that you neither enjoy doing nor have to do. For the remainder of your life, forget the different activities in category 3. Most women feel that they never get done in a day what should be done. If you eliminate category 3 and focus on the things that you enjoy doing and the things that you have to do, then you will be able to decrease your stress significantly.

Claim These Biblical
Promises For Yourself:

So don't worry about tomorrow.
—MATTHEW 6:34

You will keep in perfect peace all who trust in you, whose thoughts are fixed on you!
—ISAIAH 26:3

Give all your worries and cares to God, for he cares about what happens to you.
—1 PETER 5:7

Jesus said, "Come to me, all of you who are weary and carry heavy burdens, and I will give you rest."

—MATTHEW 11:28

Too often we try to carry our own burdens when the Lord wants to carry them for us. When we are led by the Lord, we can release the activities we should not be doing, and we can have the energy to do the things He desires for us to do. Reducing stress by giving Him your burdens will dramatically lessen the symptoms of pre-menopause or menopause.

Embrace Your Season

By applying faith to every curve and bump along the way, you can make it through this transition with grace and peace and enter into the wonderful things that God has waiting for you in the autumn season of your life. Keep learning, and keep looking to Him for guidance. This season in your life will be the best one yet. With faith in God, you cannot fail!

A BIBLE CURE PRAYER
FOR YOU

Heavenly Father, give me grace to look to You throughout all the seasons of my life, even during times of great change. I give You all my doubts, fears, concerns and cares. I thank You that You love me deeply, and You care about all that I'm going through. Help me to see Your hand in this time of my life, and help me to embrace all that You have for me. Let me be filled with Your grace during this autumn season of my life—and let it be the loveliest season of all.

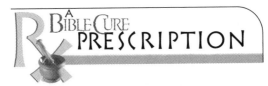

A BIBLE CURE PRESCRIPTION

List what you are doing now to reduce the stress in your life:

_____

_____

_____

_____

Now apply the following faith builder to your life, putting your name in the blanks:

Faith Builder

_____, don't worry about anything; instead, _____, pray about everything. _____, tell God what you need, and thank Him for all He has done.

—ADAPTED FROM PHILIPPIANS 4:6

A PERSONAL NOTE

From Don and Mary Colbert

God desires to heal you of disease. His Word is full of promises that confirm His love for you and His desire to give you His abundant life. His desire includes more than physical health for you; He wants to make you whole in your mind and spirit as well through a personal relationship with His Son, Jesus Christ.

If you haven't met my best friend, Jesus, I would like to take this opportunity to introduce Him to you. It is very simple.

If you are ready to let Him come into your heart and become your best friend, just bow your head and sincerely pray this prayer from your heart:

Lord Jesus, I want to know You as my Savior and Lord. I believe You are the Son of God and that You died for my sins. I also believe You were raised from the dead and now sit at the right hand of the Father praying for me. I ask You to forgive me for my sins and change my heart so that I can

be Your child and live with You eternally.
Thank You for Your peace. Help me to
walk with You so that I can begin to know
You as my best friend and my Lord. Amen.

If you have prayed this prayer, we rejoice with you in your decision and your new relationship with Jesus. Please contact us at pray4me@strang.com so that we can send you some materials that will help you become established in your relationship with the Lord. You have just made the most important decision of your life. We look forward to hearing from you.

Notes

Chapter 2
Embracing Change With Natural Hormones

1. Marcus Laux and Christine Conrad, *Natural Women, Natural Menopause* (New York: HarperCollins, 1998).
2. "Early Flash Points," *Time Magazine,* April 21, 1997, vol. 149, no. 1165 (www.time.com).

Chapter 3
Embracing Change With Healthy Nutrition

1. Margaret Lock, *Psychosomatic Medicine* (July-August 1999) as cited by Doctor's Guide (www.pslgroup.com).
2. Selene Yeager, *New Foods for Healing* (Emmaus, PA: Rodale Press, 1998), 492.

Chapter 4
Embracing Change
With Vitamins and Supplements

1. Yeager, *New Foods for Healing,* 351.

Don Colbert, M.D., was born in Tupelo, Mississippi. He attended Oral Roberts School of Medicine in Tulsa, Oklahoma, where he received a bachelor of science degree in biology in addition to his degree in medicine. Dr. Colbert completed his internship and residency with Florida Hospital in Orlando, Florida. He is board certified in family practice and has received extensive training in nutritional medicine.

If you would like more
information about natural and
divine healing, or information about
Divine Health Nutritional Products®,
you may contact
Dr. Colbert at:

DR. DON COLBERT

1908 Boothe Circle
Longwood, FL 32750
Telephone: 407-331-7007

Dr. Colbert's website is
www.drcolbert.com.

Pick up these other Siloam Press
books by Dr. Colbert:

Toxic Relief
Walking in Divine Health
What You Don't Know May Be Killing You

The Bible Cure® Booklet Series

The Bible Cure for ADD and Hyperactivity
The Bible Cure for Allergies
The Bible Cure for Arthritis
The Bible Cure for Cancer
The Bible Cure for Candida and Yeast Infection
The Bible Cure for Chronic Fatigue and Fibromyalgia
The Bible Cure for Depression and Anxiety
The Bible Cure for Diabetes
The Bible Cure for Headaches
The Bible Cure for Heart Disease
The Bible Cure for Heartburn and Indigestion
The Bible Cure for High Blood Pressure
The Bible Cure for Memory Loss
The Bible Cure for Menopause
The Bible Cure for Osteoporosis
The Bible Cure for PMS and Mood Swings
The Bible Cure for Sleep Disorders
The Bible Cure for Weight Loss and Muscle Gain

SILOAM PRESS

A part of Strang Communications Company
600 Rinehart Road
Lake Mary, FL 32746
(800) 599-5750